Welcome to my fitness training book.

I have put together this book to help you fit exercise in with your busy life and make it something you enjoy. Everyone can become fit and healthy with the right guidance so I hope you find this book useful and it puts you on track to a fitter and healthier you!

Jx

Contents

Training

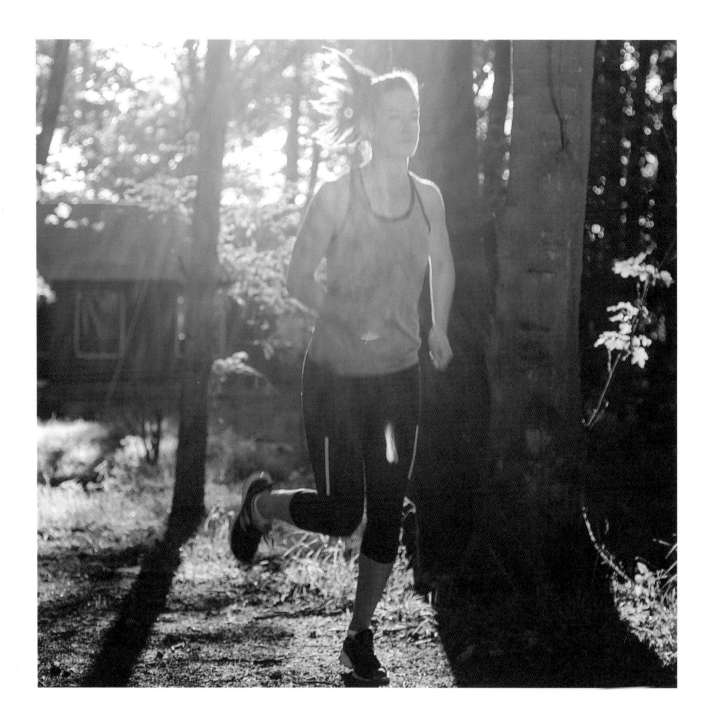

All about HIIT

This book contains a fitness training programme that runs over 12 weeks; the routines in this programme are based around HIIT – high intensity interval training, along with some cardio work.

This type of training is hard work but can be crammed into a small amount of time and therefore fit in with any lifestyle...so no excuses! With your fitness work, it is important to bear in mind that, the more you put in, the more you get out; if you work hard and give this training 100% you will see twice as much improvement than if you only give it 50%, makes sense right!

HIIT stands for short bursts of high intensity exercises with periods of rest or active recovery in between; it is designed to elevate the heart rate and really push the body to work hard, whether this is in a 10-minute workout or for a full hour.

The Benefits of HIIT

HIIT is designed to speed up your metabolism as well as to burn calories; but the element of improving metabolism is what separates HIIT from regular training.

Muscle is what's known as metabolically active tissue, meaning this is where energy and calories are burned during exercise as well as every day activities. The body has the ability to adapt to certain situations if it is placed in them regularly, such as running 5km every day. After time, the body will learn that it is running that far and conserves its energy or becomes more efficient as it becomes better trained, which, when trying to lose body fat, is the exact opposite of what we want to do! We want to be energy 'inefficient' and burn as many calories as possible and the magic of HIIT is that it is so varied, the body is left a little confused and therefore can't adapt the same, meaning it continues to burn lots of calories. It combines aerobic, anaerobic and fat burning into one workout, improving many aspects of fitness as well as the added bonus of burning calories long after your workout has finished!

As you start to lose body fat, you will also reveal your newly defined muscles. The training in your programme includes cardio and resistance training and tries to work as many areas of the body as possible; this combination will leave you with a leaner, toned looking body. Your newly revealed muscles also have benefits to your continued fat loss; you will have gained some new muscle during your training, and as I stated earlier, this is metabolically active tissue, so the more we have, the more calories we will burn at rest as well as when exercising.

Picture the body as a car, with the muscles as the engine; we will fuel the engine with body fat. If the engine is small, we will use very little fuel, meaning we won't burn much fat, but if the engine is bigger, we will need more fat to fuel it. That is why it is good to measure the changes in your body by taking body fat measurements and waist / hip circumferences rather than weighing yourself, as you may seem to remain the same weight or become slightly heavier as the muscle you have weighs more than fat.

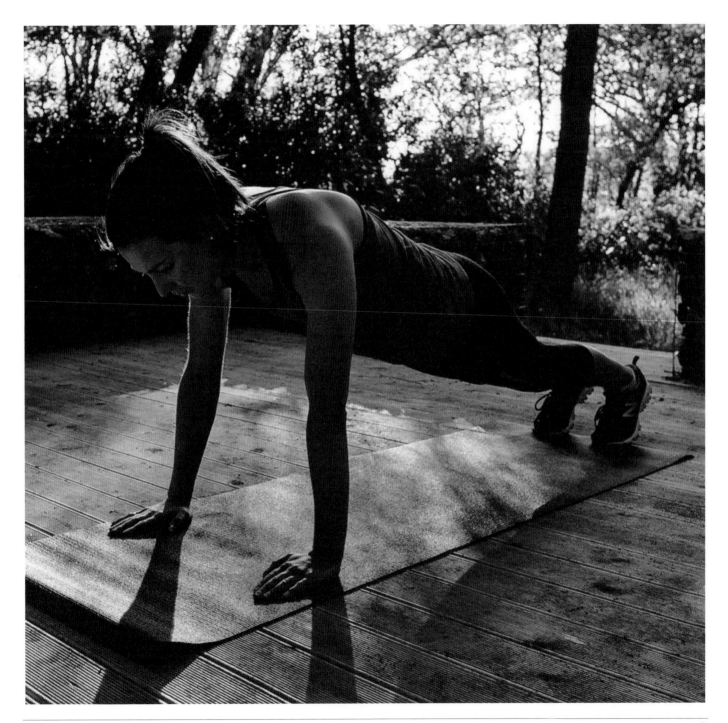

The Results

The exercises in these routines are those that will help define and tone all different areas of the body. The aim of the training is to give you a figure that you are proud of, that your clothes sit well on and that is strong but not 'bulky'.

You will be aiming to 'feel the burn', if you don't ever feel this burn, chances are you're not working hard enough! As a guide to test if you are working hard enough, ask yourself, "if someone asked you a question, would you be able to answer?"

The answer to this should be no, you should be out of breath and working to your maximum effort.

The added benefits...

Not only will HIIT help you tone up and lose body fat, it will also:

o Help strengthen bones, muscles, joints and tendons

o Improve your coordination and the body's ability to move around and control the muscles.

o Help improve heart health – the combination of aerobic and anaerobic exercises mean your heart will be getting a good work out! It is a muscle and will therefore become stronger as you train it.

o Not only will this training help improve you physically, but it will also have a positive effect on you mentally. It will teach you to push on when you are struggling, overcome hurdles that you would never usually come across and also be extremely rewarding when you see the results of your hard work.

Fitness testing

Before beginning the programme, it's good to have some starting measurements so you can monitor your progress. The body fat test provides a rough guide to your body composition. By the end of the programme you should be able to notice an improvement in your body composition as well as your fitness. If you don't want to work out your body fat, other good ways to monitor your progress include taking measurements, waist, hips etc. or by taking a 'before' picture and some progress ones every month or so.

Body Fat Percentage

This book is designed to work on reducing body fat and toning the body, due to the nature of the exercises, you will gain some muscle mass whilst losing body fat. Because muscle weighs more than fat, it is possible that you will become heavier, but this is not a bad thing! The new muscle you will have gained will help burn up more fat and also make you look more toned and defined, so you can show of a new sleek figure as you lose fat.

To work out what percentage of your body is fat and what is lean mass (bone, muscle, water etc.) you will need to take a few measurements.

Waist: Place the tape measure around the narrowest part of your abdomen, usually a few inches above the belly button and make sure the tape measure is level. Round the measurement to the nearest half inch.

Hips: Place the tape measure around the largest part of your glutes (bum) and measure the circumference, again making sure the tape measure is level and rounding to the nearest half inch.

Neck: Measure around the neck just below the larynx (Adam's apple), make sure you are stood up straight when taking the measurement and that the tape measure is straight. Round the measurement to the nearest half inch.

Calculating Your Body Fat

Using the measurements you took in inches, you can work out your body fat using this simple formula.

All you will need is a calculator with the 'log' function, if you do not have one, type it into your search engine and use an online one.

BFP= 163.205 x LOG (waist + hip – neck) – 97.684 x LOG (height in inches) – 78.387

Example: 163.205 x LOG (28.5 + 37.5 – 13) – 97.784 x LOG (69) – 78.387 = **23.2% Body Fat**

This means that 23.2% of the body is fat and the rest is lean body mass.

Guidelines for body fat suggest that:
Less Than 13 – Essential Fat
14-20% - Athletic
21-24% - Fit
25-30% - Acceptable
31% or higher – Overweight

Warming Up
&
Cooling Down

Why is it important to warm up and cool down?

The Warm Up...

Warming up before you exercise is extremely important, it helps prevent damage to your body and also helps you achieve the most from your workout.

The first part of the warm up I have designed is aiming to get your heart rate up, this means blood is pumped around the body faster, delivering oxygen to the muscles we are going to use, this allows the muscles to create energy in the cells and they will also become warm, so you are less likely to injure the muscles.

The second part of the warm up is to gently stretch the muscles and loosen them up before they do any intense work, this phase includes dynamic stretches, again meaning the muscles are less likely to become injured during the workout.

The Warm Up

Work through these warm up exercises before starting your training session.

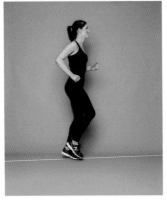

Jogging on the spot
1 Minute

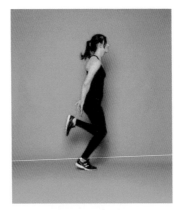

Bum kicks
30 secs

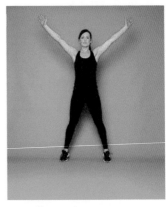

Star Jumps
30 secs

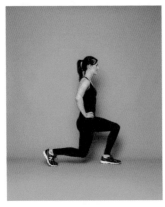

Lunges
30 secs

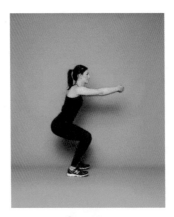

Squats
30 secs

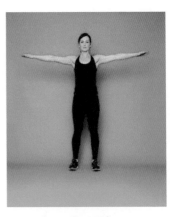

Arm Rotations
30 secs

The Cool Down...

The cooling down phase is also important and should not be missed out.
I like to include a variety of static stretches in my cool downs, working through the whole body. Stretching helps return the muscles to their original length; during exercise the muscles shorten so it is important to stretch them back out, otherwise you will end up with short tight muscles that can become damaged and also contribute to poor posture.
The cool down also helps with improving flexibility, aim to hold your stretches for about 15 seconds if you are just trying to maintain your flexibility, or if you would like to work on improving your flexibility, aim to hold them for at least 30 secs.

The Cool Down

Work through these cool down stretches after your training session.

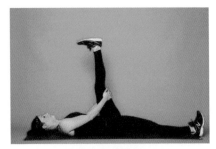

Lying Hamstring
15-30sec

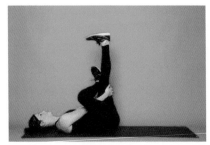

Lying Glute
15-30sec

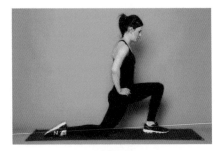

Hip Stretch
15-30sec

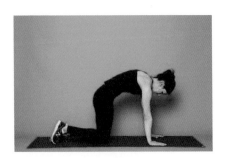

Cat Arch
15-30sec

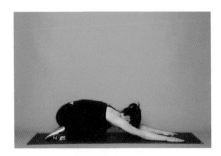

Childs Pose
15-30sec

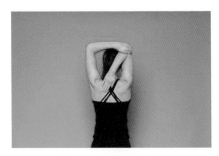

Tricep stretch
15-30sec

12 Week Training Plan

The 12 weeks ahead...

The next section of the book contains 12 weeks of training programmes.
Each week there will be a mixture of different exercises and types of training, and over the weeks the training will gradually become harder.
You can choose when you want to do each session during the week so it can fit in with your daily plans but the aim is to train once a day, 5-6 days of the week.

The HIIT sessions:

Each week there will be 2 or 3 HIIT sessions, follow the instructions on each page for each HIIT session. You will find the exercise descriptions at the back of the book.

The Cardio sessions:

There are a few different ways you can complete your cardio sessions, you will be doing two of these sessions every week and can be done outside or in the gym.
-Rowing machine / Upright cycle / Elliptical trainer
45 mins - one-hour steady pace, you shouldn't be out of breath and should be able to hold a conversation but should be sweating and hot. If you are finding you are not getting warm, add some more resistance on.
- Treadmill
45 mins - one hour, either full incline walking or steady pace jogging. you shouldn't be out of breath and should be able to hold a conversation but should be sweating and hot
- Outdoors
45mins - gentle jogging, brisk walking or cycling. You shouldn't be out of breath and should be able to hold a conversation but should be sweating and hot

The speed play sessions-

You will come across these further into the programme, if you can't fit this session in you will have the option of doing one of the HIIT sessions from earlier. These sessions again can be done outdoors or at the gym.

You can choose from jogging, cycling or rowing and this session will last 20 minutes.

You will complete one minute of light intensity (60% of your full effort).

Then 30 seconds of moderate intensity (80% of your full effort).

Then finally 30 seconds of high intensity (90-100% of your full effort).

Repeat this 10 times and remember the more you put in, the more you get from it!

Week 1

2 Long Slow Cardio Sessions
Plus
HIIT 1a, 1b and 1c

Pick one session per day
For example,
Monday – Cardio session
Tuesday- HIIT 1a
Wednesday- HIIT 1b
Thursday- Rest
Friday- Cardio session
Saturday- HIIT 1c
Sunday- Rest

HIIT Sessions
Complete each exercise one after the other.
Unless stated, only rest when all four are completed.
Rest for 30 sec. Complete this 5 times

TIP- If you can't manage the full
press ups yet, don't worry!
Just swap them for box press ups instead,
then have a go at full ones again in a couple of weeks!

HIIT 1A

Exercise	Work Time
Squat	20 sec
Star Jumps	20 sec
Plank	20 sec
Reverse Lunge	20 sec

HIIT 1B

Exercise	Work Time
Star Squat	30 sec
Heel Taps	30 sec
Lateral Lunges	30 sec
Sprint	30 sec

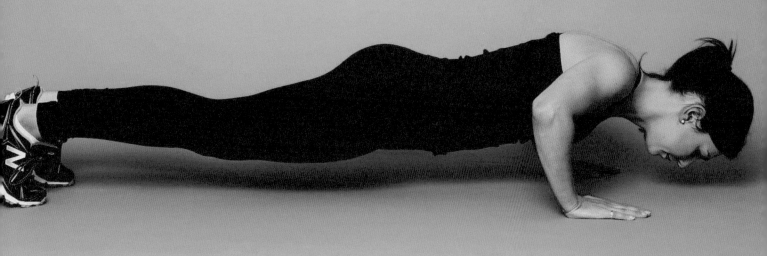

HIIT 1C

Exercise	Work Time	Rest Time
Reverse sit up	30 sec	10 sec
Squat	30 sec	10 sec
Press Up	30 sec	10 sec
Plank	30 sec	10 sec

Week 2

2 Long Slow Cardio Sessions
Plus
HIIT 1d, 1e and 1f

HIIT Sessions

Complete each exercise one
after the other. Unless stated, only rest
when all exercises are completed.
Rest for 30 sec. Complete this 5 times.

TIP- If you have any little hand weights,
kettlebells or any other weights, add them in to
increase the intensity of your workout!

HIIT 1D

Exercise	Work Time
Sprint	20 sec
Star Squat	20 sec
Burpee	20 sec
Side step touch down	20 sec
Squat Jump	20 sec

HIIT 1E

Exercise	Work Time
Mountain climber	30 sec
Star squat	30 sec
Leg swing & switch	30 sec
Burpee	30 sec
High knees & punch	30sec

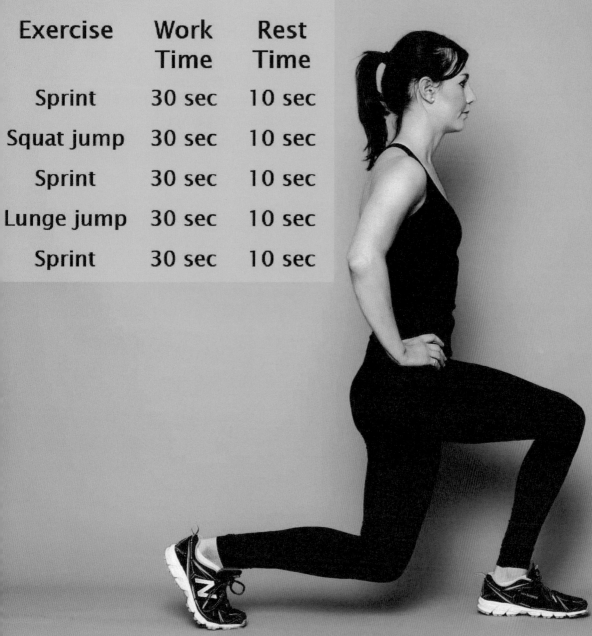

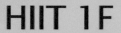

HIIT 1F

Exercise	Work Time	Rest Time
Sprint	30 sec	10 sec
Squat jump	30 sec	10 sec
Sprint	30 sec	10 sec
Lunge jump	30 sec	10 sec
Sprint	30 sec	10 sec

Week 3

2 Long Slow Cardio Sessions
Plus
HIIT 1g, 1h and 1i

HIIT Sessions

Complete each exercise one after the other.
Unless stated, only rest when all exercises are completed.
Rest for 30 sec. Complete this 5 times

HIIT 1G

Exercise	Work Time	Rest Time
Plank	20 sec	10 sec
Cross reach	20 sec	10 sec
Plank	20 sec	10 sec
Side crunch (right)	20 sec	10 sec
Plank	20 sec	10 sec
Side crunch (left)	20 sec	10 sec
Plank	20 sec	10 sec

HIIT 1H

Exercise	Work Time
Press up	30 sec
Tricep dip	30 sec
Commando plank	30 sec
Raised toe reach	30 sec
Plank punch	30 sec
Bicycle crunch	30 sec
Press up & reach	30 sec

Rest on your elbows and toes, keep the body very flat and hold this

HIIT 1I

Exercise	Work Time	Rest Time
Squat	30 sec	10 sec
Reverse lunge	30 sec	10 sec
Cross reach	30 sec	10 sec
Squat hold	30 sec	10 sec
Lunge	30 sec	10 sec
Ice skater	30 sec	10 sec
Squat hold	30 sec	10 sec

Week 4

2 Long Slow Cardio Sessions
Plus
HIIT 2a, 2b and 2c

HIIT Sessions

Complete each exercise one after the other.
Unless stated, only rest when all exercises are completed.
Rest for 30 sec. Complete this 5 times

HIIT 2A

Exercise	Work Time
Burpee	30 sec
Knee to elbow (Right)	30 sec
Mountain climbers	30 sec
Star squat	30 sec
Cross reach	30 sec
Knee to elbow (Left)	30 sec
Side crunches	30 sec

HIIT 2B

Exercise	Work Time
Cross reach	30 sec
Side crunch (R)	30 sec
Knee to elbow (R)	30 sec
Side crunch (L)	30 sec
Knee to elbow (L)	30 sec
V-up	30 sec

HIIT 2C

Exercise	Work Time
Squat jump	30 sec
Lunge jump	30 sec
Lateral lunges (R)	30 sec
Scissor squat	30 sec
Lateral lunges (L)	30 sec
Star squat	30 sec
Press up & reach	30 sec
Bicycle crunch	30 sec

Week 5

2 Long Slow Cardio Sessions
Plus
1 speed play session
plus
HIIT 2d and 2e

HIIT Sessions

Complete each exercise for 30 seconds one after the other until you have completed the set (A,B,C or D). Rest for 30 sec. Complete each set 3 times before moving onto the next.

HIIT 2d

Exercise	Work Time
SET A Tuck star Knees to squat stance High knees punch Courtesy lunge	30 sec
SET B Sprint Reverse sit up Press up & knee raise Star press	30 sec
SET C Squat jump Lateral legs Mountain climbers V-up	30 sec
SET D Knee to elbow (R) Russian twist Knee to elbow (L) Plank	30 sec

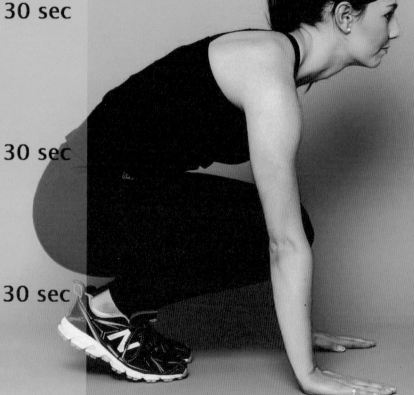

HIIT 2e

Exercise	Work Time
SET A Burpee Swing & switch Star squat High knees punch	30 sec
SET B Side plank crunch (R) Lunge jump Side plank crunch (L) Sprint	30 sec
SET C Press up & knee raise Squat raise (R) Ice skater Squat raise (L)	30 sec
SET D Spiderman plank Side crunch (R) Rowing boat Side crunch (L)	30 sec

Week 6

2 Long Slow Cardio Sessions
Plus
HIIT 2f, 2g and 2h

HIIT Sessions

Complete each exercise one after the other.
Unless stated, only rest when all exercises are completed.
Rest for 30 sec. Complete this 5 times

HIIT 2f

Exercise	Work Time
Burpee	30 sec
Plank punch	30 sec
Burpee	30 sec
Squat hold	30 sec
Burpee	30 sec
Scissor squat	30 sec
Burpee	30 sec

HIIT 2g

Exercise	Work Time
High knees punch	30 sec
Squat jump	30 sec
Press up & knee raise	30 sec
Lunge jump	30 sec
Cross reach	30 sec
Squat star	30 sec
Spiderman plank	30 sec

HIIT 2h

Exercise	Work Time	Rest Time
Plank	45 sec	15 sec
Press up & reach	45 sec	15 sec
Plank punch	45 sec	15 sec
Star press	45 sec	15 sec
Spiderman plank	45 sec	15 sec
Tricep dip	45 sec	15 sec
Russian twist	45 sec	15 sec

Week 7

2 Long Slow Cardio Sessions
Plus
1 speed play session
plus
HIIT 3a and 3b

HIIT Sessions

Complete each set (starting with A, B then C) 3 times, only resting for the stated 10 seconds until the set is completed 3 times. After the 3rd completion, rest for 30 seconds, then move onto the next set.

HIIT 3a

Exercise	Work Time	Rest Time
SET A Sprint Squat jump Lunge jump Swing & switch	30 sec	10 sec
SET B Press up & reach Tricep dip Commando plank Press up & knee raise	30 sec	10 sec
SET C Rowing boat Reverse sit up Russian twist Spiderman plank	30 sec	10 sec

HIIT 3b

Exercise	Work Time	Rest Time
SET A		
High knees punch		
Bear crawl	30	10
Seated squat	sec	sec
thrust		
Burpee		
SET B		
Mountain climber		
Side crunch (R)	30	10
Plank punch	sec	sec
Side crunch (L)		
SET C		
Cross reach		
V–up	30	10
Side plank (R)	sec	sec
Side plank (L)		

Week 8

2 Long Slow Cardio Sessions
Plus
HIIT 3c, 3d and 3e

HIIT Sessions

Complete each exercise one after the other.
Only rest when all exercises are completed.
Rest for 30 sec. Complete this 3 times

HIIT 3c

Exercise	Work Time
Plank	30 sec
Side crunch (R)	30 sec
Bicycle crunch	30 sec
Wide/narrow plank jumps	30 sec
Reverse sit up	30 sec
Side crunch (L)	30 sec
Russian twist	30 sec
Lateral legs	30 sec

HIIT 3d

Exercise	Work Time
Sprint	30 sec
Squat hold	30 sec
High knees punch	30 sec
Swing & switch	30 sec
Burpees	30 sec
Mountain climber	30 sec
Ice skater	30 sec
Lateral lunge	30 sec

HIIT 3e

Exercise	Work Time
Star press	30 sec
Reverse flutter	30 sec
Knee to elbow (R)	30 sec
Seated squat thrust	30 sec
Knee to elbow (L)	30 sec
Reverse criss cross	30 sec
Tuck star	30 sec
Spiderman press up	30 sec

Week 9

2 Long Slow Cardio Sessions
Plus
1 Speed play session
plus
HIIT 3f and 3g

HIIT 3f

Complete each set then rest for 30 seconds.
Complete each set 3 times before moving on to the next set.

HIIT 3f

Exercise	Work Time
SET A Reverse lunge Scissor squat Ice skater High knees punch	30 sec
SET B Burpees Knee to elbow (R) Seated squat thrust Knee to elbow (L)	30 sec
SET C Squat raise (R) Tuck star Squat raise (L) Lateral legs	30 sec
SET D Star squat Bear crawl Sprint Cross reach	30 sec
SET D Press up & reach Side crunch (R) Side step touch down Side crunch (L)	30 sec

HIIT 3g

Exercise	Work Time	Active recovery / Rest	Time
SET A		*SET A*	
High knees punch	30	Squat hold	30
Press up & knee raise	sec	Plank	sec
Cross reach		Rest	
SET B		*SET B*	
Mountain climber	30	Squat hold	30
Burpee	sec	Plank	sec
Sprint		Rest	
SET C		*SET C*	
Scissor squat	30	Squat hold	30
Reverse sit up	sec	Plank	sec
Swing & switch		Rest	

Week 10

2 Long Slow Cardio Sessions
Plus
HIIT 4a, 4b and 4c

HIIT Sessions

Work through the exercises resting for 10 seconds between each one.
Repeat 3 times.

HIIT 4a

Exercise	Work Time	Rest Time
High knees punch	30 sec	10 sec
Squat jump	30 sec	10 sec
High knees punch	30 sec	10 sec
Spiderman press up	30 sec	10 sec
High knees punch	30 sec	10 sec
Reverse criss cross	30 sec	10 sec
High knees punch	30 sec	10 sec
Reverse flutter		

HIIT 4b

Exercise	Work Time	Rest Time
Bear crawl & press up	30 sec	10 sec
Tricep dip	30 sec	10 sec
W/N plank jump	30 sec	10 sec
Spiderman burpee	30 sec	10 sec
Mountain climbers	30 sec	10 sec
Lunge jump	30 sec	10 sec
Side plank crunch (R)	30 sec	10 sec
Reverse Plank	30 sec	10 sec
Side plank crunch (L)	30 sec	10 sec
Plank toe taps	30 sec	10 sec

HIIT 4c

Exercise	Work Time	Rest Time
Sprint	30 sec	10 sec
Swing & switch	30 sec	10 sec
Seated squat thrust	30 sec	10 sec
Single leg plank (R)	30 sec	10 sec
Burpee & press up	30 sec	10 sec
Single leg plank (L)	30 sec	10 sec
High knees punch	30 sec	10 sec
V-up	30 sec	10 sec
Bicycle crunch	30 sec	10 sec
Plank punch	30 sec	10 sec

Week 11

2 Long Slow Cardio Sessions
Plus
1 Speed play session
plus
HIIT 4d and 4e

HIIT Sessions
Complete each set (starting with A, B then C), resting for 1 minute when the set is complete before moving onto the next one.
Go through this twice.

HIIT 4d

SET A		SET B		SET C	
Exercise	Work Time	Exercise	Work Time	Exercise	Work Time
High knees punch	30 sec	Star press	30 sec	Mountain climber	30 sec
Bear crawl	30 sec	Press up & knee raise	30 sec	Rowing boat	30 sec
Plank toe taps	30 sec	Tricep dip	30 sec	Russian twist	30 sec
Reverse flutter	30 sec	Burpee & press up	30 sec	Side plank crunch (R)	30 sec
Seated squat thrust	30 sec	Commando plank	30 sec	Spiderman plank	30 sec
Reverse criss cross	30 sec	Sprint	30 sec	Side plank crunch (L)	30 sec

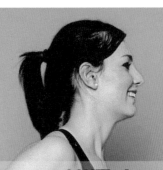

HIIT 4e

SET A		SET B		SET C	
Exercise	Work Time	Exercise	Work Time	Exercise	Work Time
Sprint	30 sec	High knees punch	30 sec	Star squat	30 sec
Star squat	30 sec	Lunge jump	30 sec	Cross reach	30 sec
Press up & reach	30 sec	Ice skater	30 sec	Sprint	30 sec
Mountain climbers	30 sec	Knee to elbow (R)	30 sec	V–up	30 sec
Swing & switch	30 sec	Squat jump	30 sec	Bicycle crunch	30 sec
Knees to squat stance	30 sec	Knee to elbow (L)	30 sec	Plank toe taps	30 sec

Week 12

2 Long Slow Cardio Sessions
Plus
HIIT 4f, 4g and 4h

HIIT 4f and 4g

Complete each exercise one after the other with a 10 sec rest between. Rest for 30 secs at the end of the set. Repeat 6 times.

HIIT 4f

Exercise	Work Time	Rest
Squat jumps	30 sec	10 sec
Mountain climbers	30 sec	10 sec
Spiderman burpee	30 sec	10 sec
Press up & knee raise	30 sec	10 sec
Side crunches	30 sec	10 sec

HIIT 4g

Exercise	Work Time	Rest
High knees punch	30 sec	10 sec
Seated squat thrust	30 sec	10 sec
Sprint	30 sec	10 sec
Tricep dips	30 sec	10 sec
Spiderman press up	30 sec	10 sec

HIIT 4h

Complete each exercise one after the other until you have completed the set (A,B,C,D,E then F). Rest for 30 sec at the end of the set, complete each set 3 times before moving onto the next.

HIIT 4h

Exercise	Work Time
SET A	
High knees punch	
Tuck star	30 sec
Mountain climbers	
Squats	
SET B	
Burpees	
Spiderman press up	30 sec
Tricep dip	
Lunge jumps	
SET C	
Swing & switch	
Seated squat thrust	30 sec
Commando plank	
Rowing boat	
SET D	
Sprint	
Squat star	30 sec
Knees to squat stance	
Plank toe taps	
SET E	
Ice skater	
Squat jump	30 sec
Side plank crunch (R)	
Side plank crunch (L)	
SET F	
Reverse flutter	
Russian twist	30 sec
Reverse criss cross	
V-up	

Exercise Descriptions

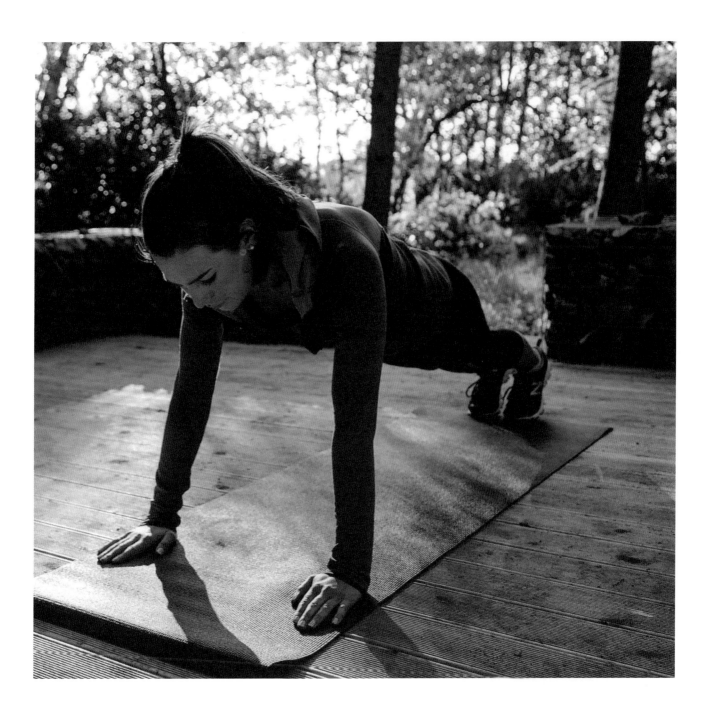

Bear Crawl

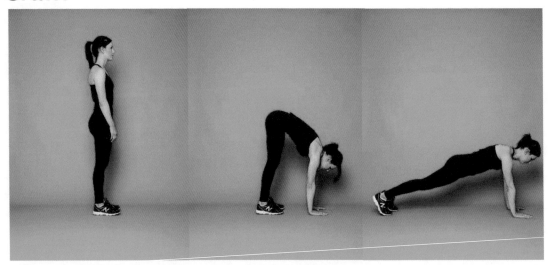

· Stand with feet hip width apart and flat on the floor
· Reach the hands down and place them flat on the floor in line with the feet (as close as you can get to the feet)
· From this position, walk your hands out until your body is flat and fully extended.
· Then walk the hands back in towards the feet and stand up straight.

Bear Crawl & Press Up

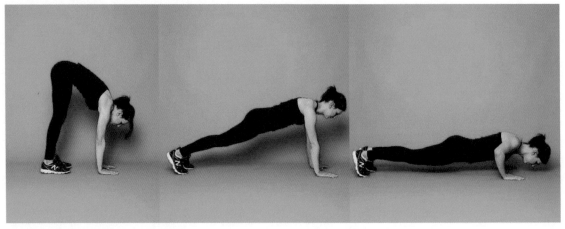

· When in the fully extended position complete a press up before walking the hands back in.

Bicycle Crunch

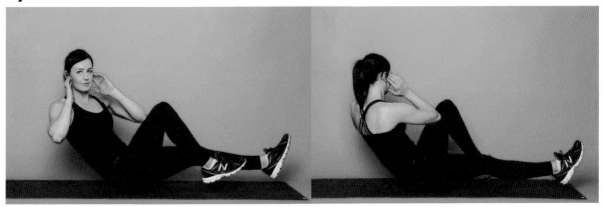

·Sit on your bum with right knee bent and the left leg out straight.
·Place the left elbow on the raised knee, then switch and bend the left leg, straighten the right leg and bring the right elbow to the left knee.
·Repeat in a rhythm.

Box Press Up

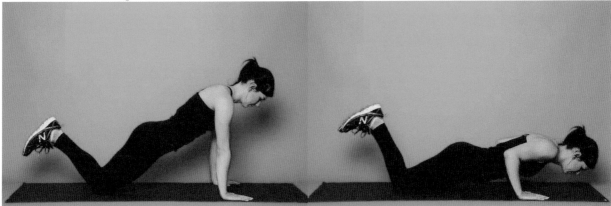

· Place your hands slightly wider than shoulder width apart at chest level
· Place your feet out behind you with legs straight to find the right position, then drop down on to your knees, raise your feet off the floor then cross them over.
· From this position, lower your chest towards the floor, bending at the elbows, then extend and push back up. Keep the back flat and core engaged

Burpee

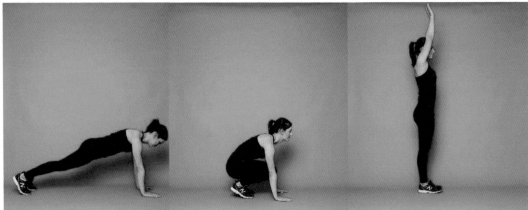

· Start in a press up position, jump your feet forward towards your hands, keeping them together.
· Then jump up and raise your arms above your head.
· Jump back to the press up start position.

Burpee & Press Up

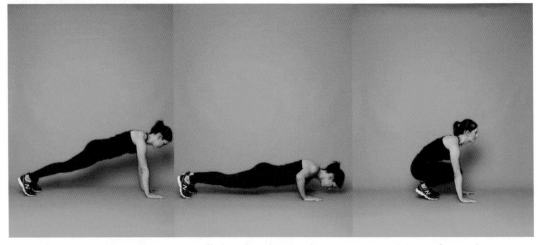

· After completing a burpee, you will be back to the start position, from here complete a full press up before performing another burpee.

Commando Plank

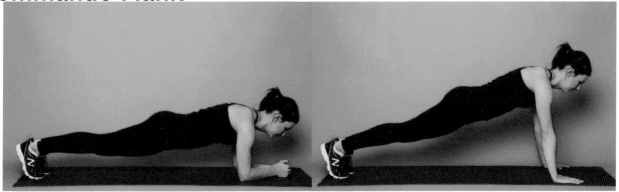

· Rest on your elbows and toes with your body flat in a regular plank position
· Push up onto your hands then lower back to the elbows, one at a time.
·Try to keep your body as still a possible.

Commando Press Up

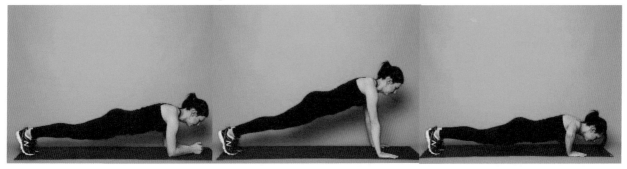

· Rest on your elbows and toes with your body flat in a regular plank position
· Push up onto your hands then complete one press up
· Lower back to the elbows, one at a time.
·Try to keep your body as still a possible.

Courtesy Lunge

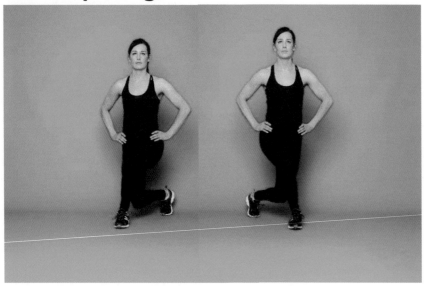

· Place hands on the hips, keep the body up tall and step one foot out behind the other and bend at both knees.
· Return the feet together and repeat for the other side.

Cross Reach

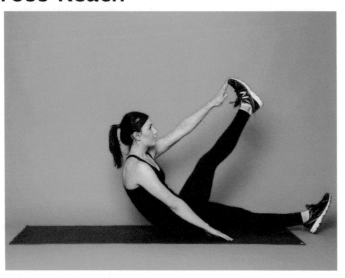

· Lie on your back with arms out flat on the floor above your head and legs out straight
· Raise one foot up, and bring the opposite hand up and to meet the toes then lower and switch legs.

Fallen Star

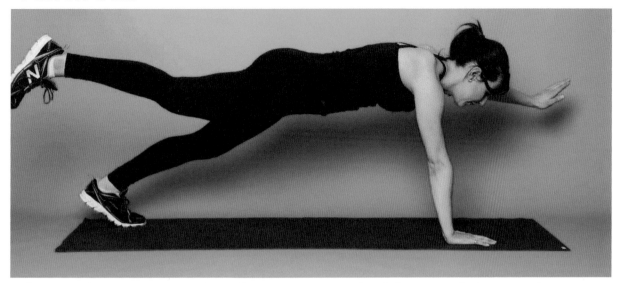

·Go into the starting position of a press up, maintaining your balance, raise one hand and the opposite foot off the floor.
·Hold for 3 seconds then return them to the floor and repeat for the other hand and foot.

Frog Jump

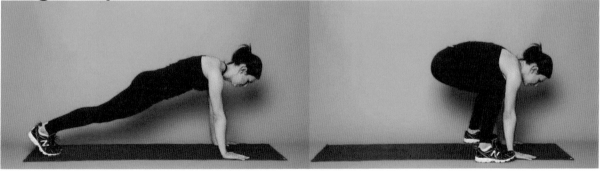

·Go into the start phase of a press up, jump both feet forward so they are next to your hands.
· Jump back to the start position, maintain a tight core throughout.

Heel Taps

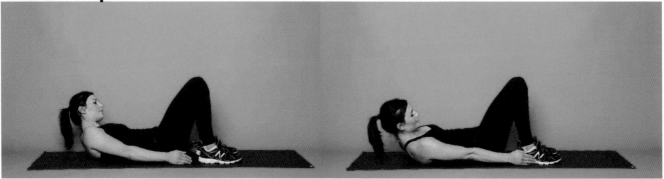

· Lie on your back with knees bent and feet flat on the floor
· Squeeze your abs to lift your shoulders off the floor slightly. Reach round with your right hand to try and touch your right heel
· Repeat with the left side, if you can't reach your heels, move your feet in towards you bum a bit more.

High Knees Punch

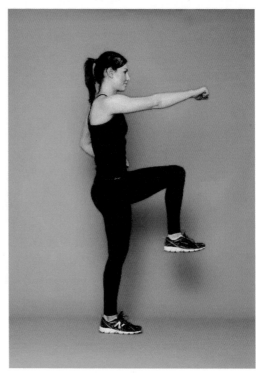

· Start running but bring the knees up as high as you can and whilst you do this, punch your arms out straight in front of you.
· Keep light on your toes and go as fast as you can on the spot, lifting your knees up as high as you can.
· Keep the core tight and the body up tall.

Ice Skater

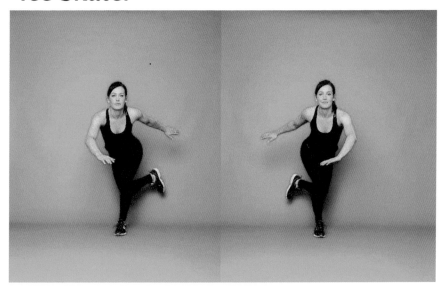

· Stand on the right foot with the left foot raised off the floor and out behind the supporting leg.
· Reach down slightly with the left hand towards the floor
· Push off the right leg and switch over your legs as your arms swing and switch over too.

Jogging On the Spot

· Keep your eyes up and body tall
· Stay light on your feet and jog on the spot at a steady pace.

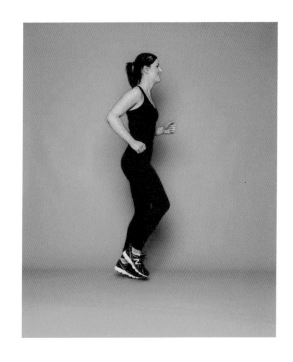

Knee to Elbow

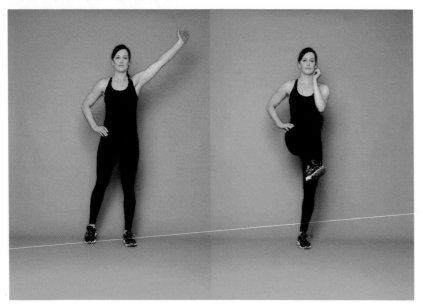

· Stand with feet slightly wider than hip width apart, raise one knee up towards the opposite elbow, crunch the abs.
· Lower the leg but keep your arm in the air, then repeat.

Knees to Squat Stance

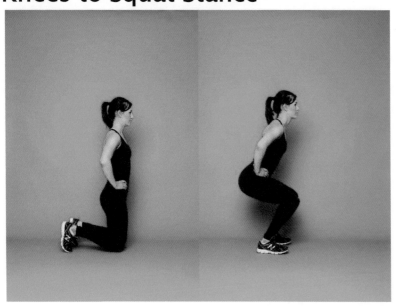

· Start on your knees with them at a 90-degree angle and your body up straight.
· From this position, step up on to your feet, but remain low and in a squat stance.
· Return to your knees and repeat.

Lateral Legs

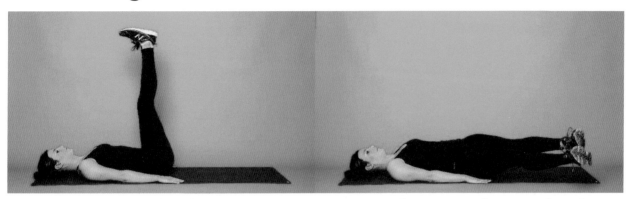

· Lie on your back with feet together; raise them together up so they are directly above your hips.
· Keeping it slow and controlled, lower the legs to alternating sides, keeping the feet together.

Lateral Lunge

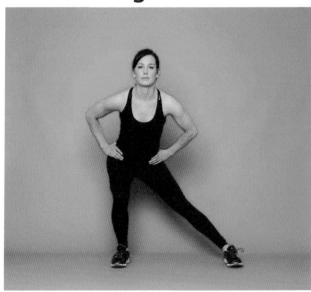

· Stand with feet together, then step out to the side and bend the knee that you have stepped out onto.
· Keep the body upright and hands on the hips.
· Step back in and repeat for the other side.

Lunge Jump

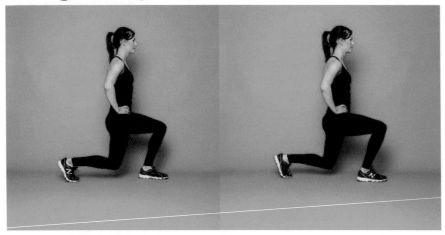

· Step one foot out in front and let the front knee bend to a 90-degree angle and the back knee drop to a 90-degree angle.
· From this position, jump up and switch the legs over and repeat.
· Keep hands on the hips and the body up.

Mountain Climbers

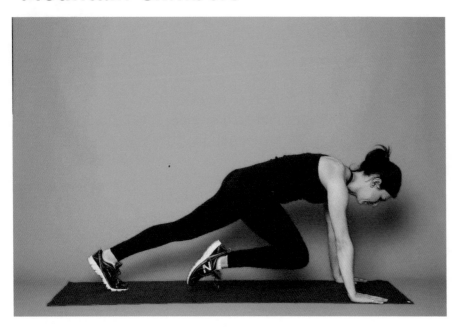

· Place the hands on the floor and place the feet in the staggered position (as if you were coming out the starting blocks in a race) with the body flat.
· Start a running action, drawing one knee at a time up towards the chest, staying light on the toes and tight through the core.

Plank

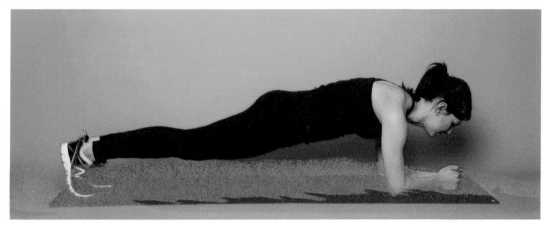

- Rest on your elbows and toes, keep the body very flat and hold this position.
- Be careful not to let the back dip or point your bum in the air.

Plank Punch

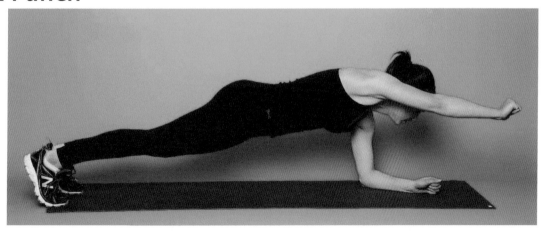

- From the plank position, punch one arm at a time out in front of you
- Try and keep the body as still and flat as possible.

Plank Toe Taps

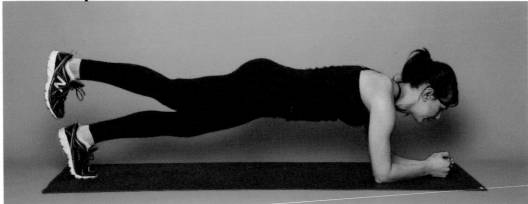

· From the plank position, squeeze the glutes (bum muscles) and raise one leg at a time off the floor.
· Keep the legs straight and make the movements small and controlled.

Press Up

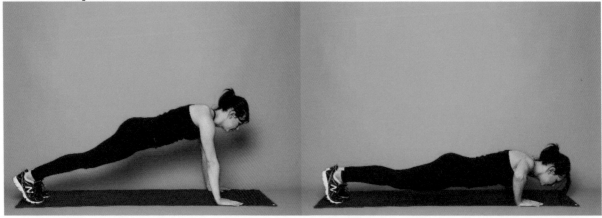

· Rest on hands and feet with arms straight and body flat.
· Bend at the elbows and lower the chest towards the floor then push back up
· For an easier option, use a box press up.

Press up and Knee Raise

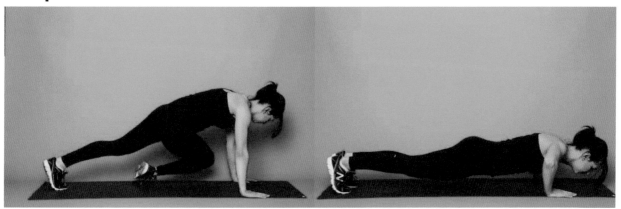

· Start in a press up position, raise one knee at a time up towards the opposite hand.
· Once you have done this for each leg complete a press up.

Press up and Reach

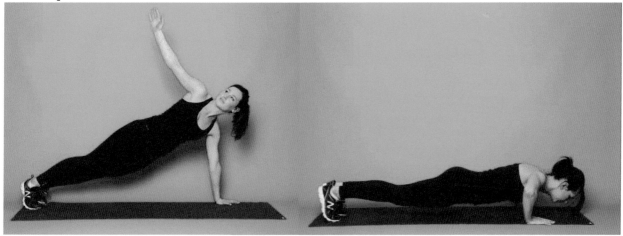

· Complete a press up then reach one arm up and point it up to the sky, follow it with your eyes, then lower back to the floor.
· Complete another press up then reach up with the other arm.

Raised Toe Reach

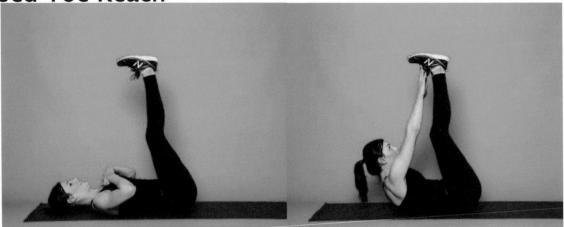

· Lie on your back and cross feet over. Raise your feet up to the sky, above the hips at a 90-degree angle.
· Reach your hands up towards your feet from your chest., squeezing your tummy muscles to raise your upper body off the floor.

Reverse Criss Cross

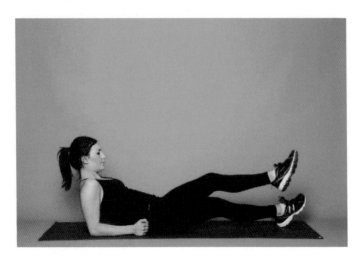

· Balance on your bum with legs straight and slightly raised off the floor. Position your elbows on the floor behind you to support yourself.
· Cross the feet over, switching which foot goes over the top each time.
· Keep the legs very straight and make the action very quick.

Reverse Flutter

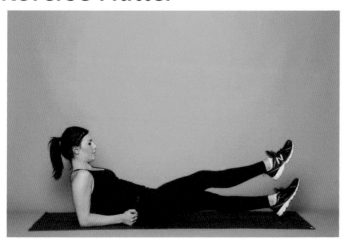

· Balance on your bum with legs straight and slightly raised off the floor. Position your elbows on the floor behind you to support yourself.
· Move the feet up and down quickly in a fluttering motion.
· Keep the legs very straight and make the action very quick.

Reverse Lunge

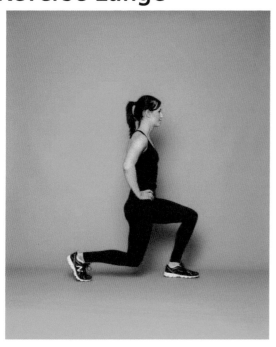

· Place hands on hips, step one foot back and drop the knee to a 90-degree angle whilst the one in the front also stays at a 90-degree angle.
· Step back up and repeat with the other leg, keeping the body tall and everything straight.

Reverse Plank

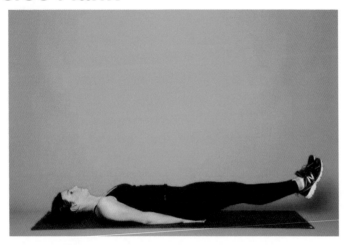

· Lie on your back (with hands under your bum if you need to)
· Raise your feet about 6 inches off the floor and hold
·Try to keep your body as flat as possible and make sure the core is engaged, taking the weight of your legs.

Reverse Sit Up

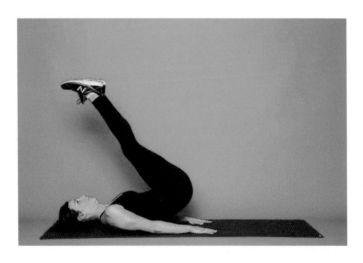

· Lie on your back with your hands under your bum and legs out straight.
· Squeeze your abs and raise your feet off the floor until they are as far up and back as you can get them, then slowly lower again.
· Keep your feet together throughout.

Rowing Boat

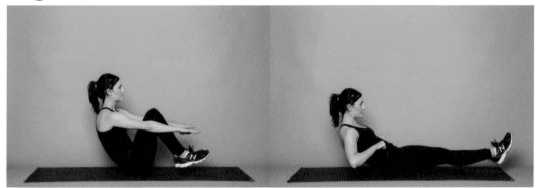

· Sit on your bum with your knees tucked in towards your chest and your arms extended next to the legs
· Extend the legs out, but don't let them touch the floor, at the same time, bend the elbows in a rowing action and lower the body slightly.
· Squeeze the abs and bring the body back up to your starting position.

Russian Twist

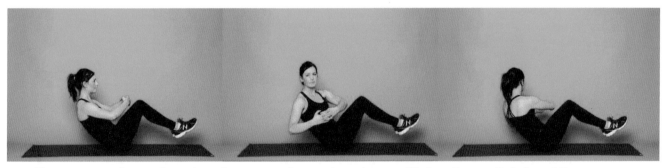

·Sit on your bum, keeping feet together raise them off the floor slightly whilst bending the knees.
· Hold your arms in an arch out in front of you and rotate from side to side, twisting through your middle.

Sandwiches

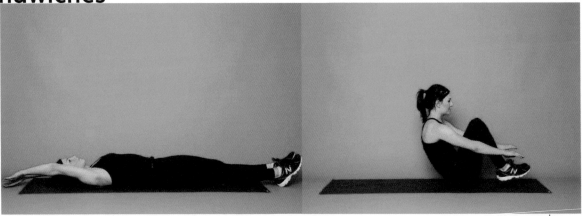

· Lie on your back with your arms out straight behind you and legs flat on the floor.
· Bring your arms over your head whilst raising the upper body off the floor and bending the knees in towards your chest.
· Keep the arms straight and down by your side, then slowly return to the start position.

Scissor Squat

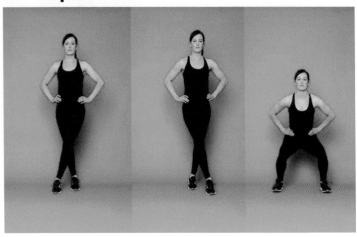

· Stand with one foot slightly in front of the other then using a jumping action, switch the feet over
· Then from this position, jump into a squat
· Then jump back to the start position.

Seated Squat Thrust

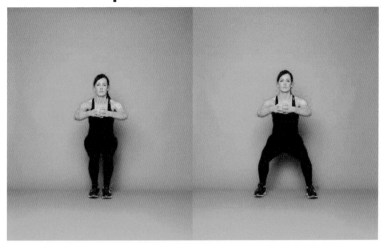

· Sit into a squat position, feet slightly wider than hip width apart and making sure the knees don't go over the toes.
· From this starting position, jump the feet in so they are together, remaining in the seated squat position.
· Jump the feet back out to the starting position, still remaining in the seated squat.

Side Crunch

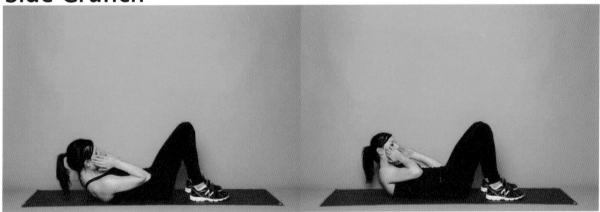

· Lie on your back with knees bent and feet flat on the floor
· Place hands by your ears and squeeze your abs to raise the upper body off the floor slightly
· Squeeze down the side of your body to bring one elbow towards the hip on that side, return to the starting position and repeat.

Side Plank

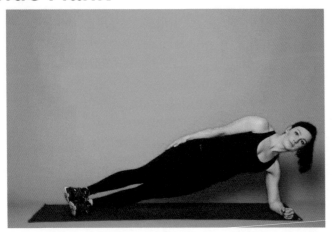

· Rest on the right elbow and the right foot, raise your hips and body off the floor.
· Hold this position and repeat for the other side·

Side Plank Crunch

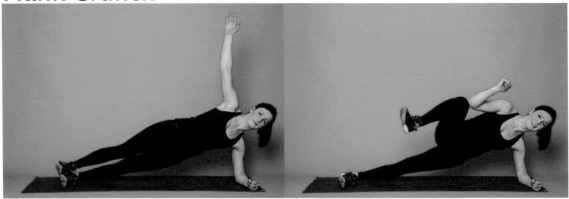

· Rest on the right elbow and the right foot, raise your hips and body off the floor.
· Start with your left arm in the air above you, then bend your left knee and elbow at the same time, drawing them together to crunch down the left side of the body.
· Straighten both the arm and the leg back out and repeat.

Side Plank Reach

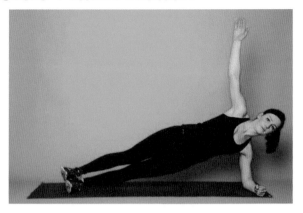

· Rest on the right elbow and the right foot, raise your hips and body off the floor.
· Start with your left arm in the air above you, then reach down and scoop it under your body.
· Reach back up again and repeat.

Side Step Touch

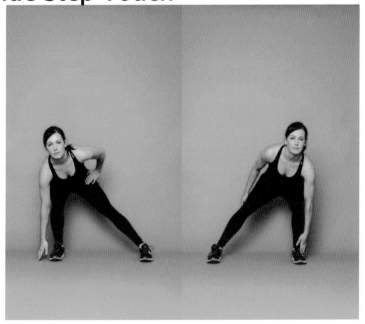

· Step over to the side by two steps, touch the floor then repeat the other way.
· Stay light on the toes and move as quickly as you can, keep the knees bent at all times.

Single Leg Plank

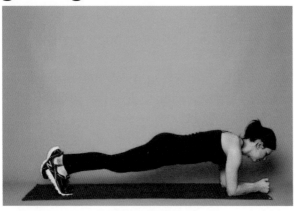

· Start in a regular plank position, then cross one leg over the other.
·Keep the body as level and flat as possible and hold this position.

Spiderman Burpee

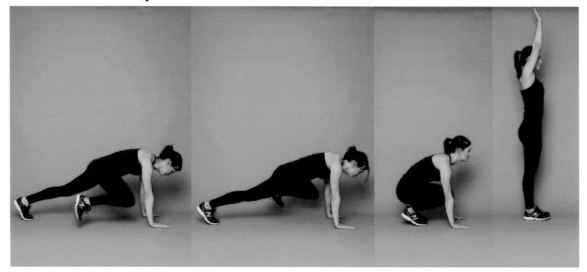

· Start in a press up position, raise one knee at a time out to the side and up towards your elbow.
· Return to start position then jump feet in towards hands and jump up raising arms above your head.

Spiderman Plank

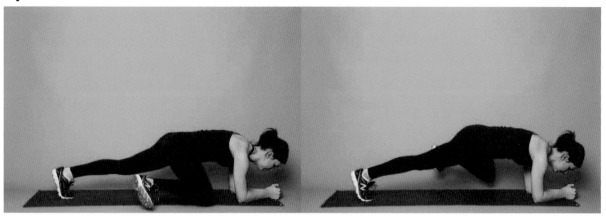

· From the plank, bring one knee at a time out to the side and up towards the elbow.
· Keep the body very flat at all times and make sure the bum doesn't point up in the air or the back doesn't start to dip.

Spiderman Press Up

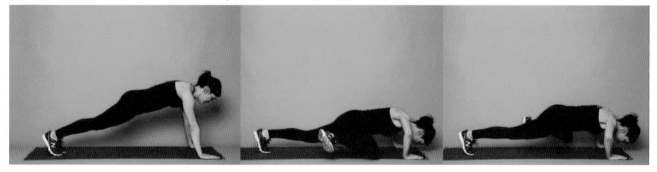

· Start in a regular press up position.
· When you go into the downwards phase of the press up, hold and bring one knee at a time out to the side and towards the elbow.
· Do this for both legs before pushing back up to the starting position.

Sprint

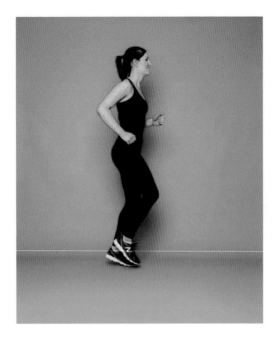

· Sprint on the spot, keeping light on the toes and the body upright.
· Push yourself to go as fast as you can.

Squat

· Stand with feet slightly wider than hip width apart
· Drop down as if you are sitting into a chair, keeping the weight in your heels, body up and arms out in front of you.

Squat Hold

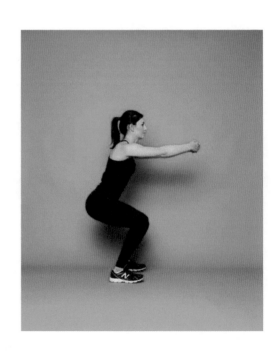

· Drop down into a squat position, keeping the weight in the heels and arms out in front.
·Hold this position.

Squat Jump

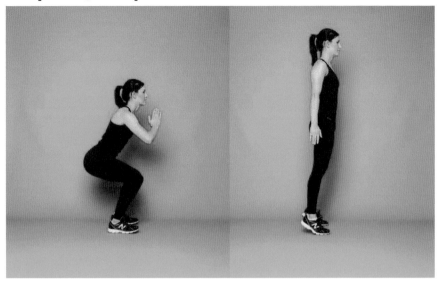

· Drop down into a squat position then push up and jump as high as you can.
· Land in the squat position and repeat.

Squat Raise

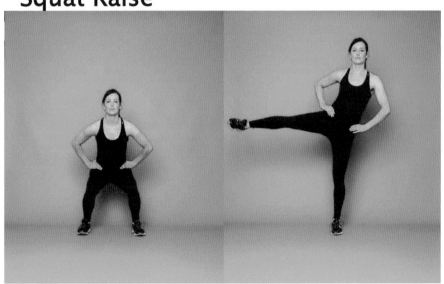

· Start in a squat position
· Stand up and raise one leg up and out to the side
· Lower back to the start position and repeat.

Star Jump

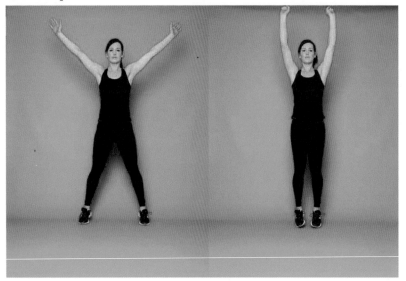

· Jump and swing the arms up above the head and the feet together.
· Jump again and place arms back down by the side and the feet slightly wider than hip width apart.

Star Press

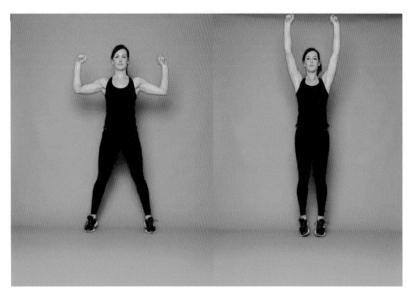

· Start with hands level with your ears and elbows bent with your feet out wide
· Jump the feet in as if completing a normal star jump, but press the hands up above your shoulders.
· Return to start position and repeat.

Star Squat

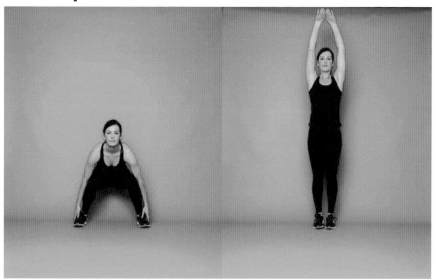

· Start in a squat position with hands down by the feet.
· Jump up and swing arms over the head and feet together
· Jump back down into the start position

Tricep Dips

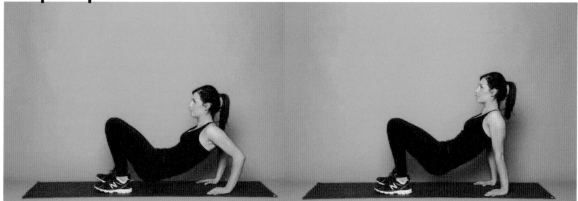

· Place hands behind you with fingers pointing towards your bum.
· Position feet in towards your bum, flat on the floor with bum raised.
· Bend the elbows and lower the body towards the floor, then straighten the elbows and raise the body up again.
· This can also be done with the hands resting on a bench or step.

Tuck Star

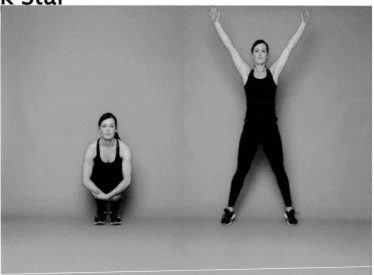

· Place both feet together and squat down to wrap your arms around the legs.
· From that position, burst up into a star jump
· Then return to the start position in a smooth motion.

V–Up

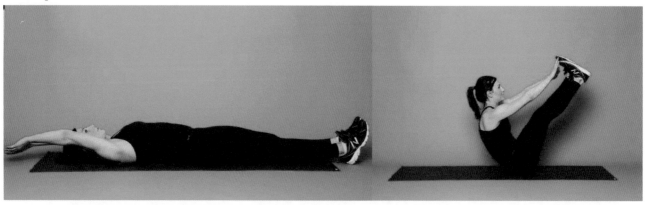

· Lie on your back with arms and legs out straight, squeeze the tummy muscles and raise both hands and feet up towards the sky and try and get them to meet in the middle above the hips.
· Slowly lower and repeat

Wide Narrow Plank Jumps

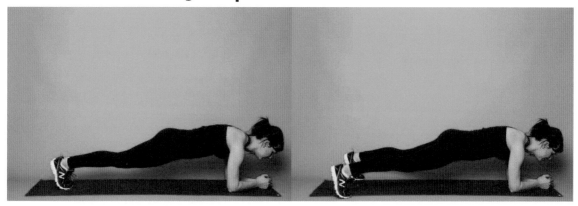

· Start in a regular plank position
· Keeping the body flat, jump the feet out wide then back to the start position
· Repeat, keeping the body very flat and legs straight

Index of Exercises

The exercises and training programmes have been designed with care but are completed at the readers own risk. The author cannot accept any responsibility for any injuries suffered as a result of completing exercises outlined in this book and disclaim any responsibility for loss, liability, risk, personal or otherwise as a consequence of using this book either directly or indirectly.
The ideas in this book may aid in improving fitness but does not replace the advice of health care professionals and it is recommended that you consult a physician before starting any exercise programme.

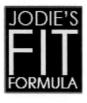

A special thanks to Matt Brown and Lizzy Coates for their help with this book.

Printed in Great Britain
by Amazon